Hypothyroidism Cookbook

**MAIN COURSE – Hypothyroidism
Breakfast, Lunch, Dinner and Dessert
Recipes**

TABLE OF CONTENTS

part of this document in either electronic means or in printed format. Recording of this publication is strictly prohibited and any storage of this document is not allowed unless with written permission from the publisher. All rights reserved.

The information provided herein is stated to be truthful and consistent, in that any liability, in terms of inattention or otherwise, by any usage or abuse of any policies, processes, or directions contained within is the solitary and utter responsibility of the recipient reader. Under no circumstances will any legal responsibility or blame be held against the publisher for any reparation, damages, or monetary loss due to the information herein, either directly or indirectly.

Respective authors own all copyrights not held by the publisher.

The information herein is offered for informational purposes solely, and is universal as so. The presentation of the information is without contract or any type of guarantee assurance.

The trademarks that are used are without any consent, and the publication of the trademark is without permission or backing by the trademark owner. All trademarks and brands within this book are for clarifying purposes only and are the owned by the owners themselves, not affiliated with this document.

Introduction

Hypothyroidism recipes for personal enjoyment but also for family enjoyment. You will love them for sure for how easy it is to prepare them.

MILK QUINOA PORRIDGE

Serves: *1*

Prep Time: *5*   Minutes

Cook Time: *5*   Minutes

Total Time: *10*   Minutes

INGREDIENTS

- 1 cup quinoa
- 1 cup unsweetened coconut milk
- 1 tsp vanilla extract
- 1 tsp turmeric
- 1 tsp cinnamon
- ¼ tsp salt
- ¼ cup raisins
- ½ cup coconut flakes

DIRECTIONS

1. In your instant pot add quinoa and coconut milk and whisk well
2. Set to high pressure and cook for 2-3 minutes, allow to rest

3. Remove the lid an add the rest of the ingredients, top with coconut flakes
4. Serve when ready

Serves: *4*
Prep Time: *10* Minutes

Cook Time: *30* Minutes

Total Time: *40* Minutes

INGREDIENTS

- 1 cup rolled oats
- 4 tablespoons urad dal
- 4 tsp ghee
- salt

DIRECTIONS

1. In a blender add oats, urad dal and blend until smooth
2. Add water and blend again
3. Transfer the mixture to a bowl and set aside overnight
4. Add salt, mix well and pour the mixture in a skillet and cook for 4-5 minutes per side
5. When ready remove from heat and serve

Serves: *1*
Prep Time: **5**   Minutes

Cook Time: **5**   Minutes

Total Time: **10**   Minutes

INGREDIENTS

- 1 cup strawberries
- ¼ cup coconut sugar
- 1 cup coconut milk
- Mint leaves

DIRECTIONS

1. In a blender add all ingredients and blend until smooth
2. When ready, serve with mint leaves

Serves: **6**

Prep Time: **5** Minutes

Cook Time: **15** Minutes

Total Time: **20** Minutes

INGREDIENTS

- ¼ cup oats
- ¼ cup onions whites
- ¼ cup urad dal
- 1 tsp black pepper
- 1 tsp olive oil

DIRECTIONS

1. Blend the urad dal until smooth
2. Transfer mixture to a bowl, add the rest of the ingredients and mix well
3. Pour the batter into an appe mold and cook until they are done
4. When ready remove from heat and serve

Serves: *6*
Prep Time: *5*   Minutes

Cook Time: *10*   Minutes

Total Time: *15*   Minutes

INGREDIENTS

- 1 cup buckwheat
- ¼ cup low fat curds
- 1 tsp chilli paste
- 1 tablespoon coriander
- Pinch of turmeric powder
- Salt
- 1 tsp olive oil

DIRECTIONS

1. In a bowl combine all ingredients together
2. In a skillet heat olive oil and pour 1/6 cup of the batter
3. Cook for 1-2 minutes per side
4. When ready remove from heat and serve

Serves: *1*

Prep Time: *5*   Minutes

Cook Time: *5*   Minutes

Total Time: *10*   Minutes

INGREDIENTS

- 2 egg whites
- 1 tsp olive oil
- Salt
- ¼ cup onions
- ¼ cup yellow capsicum
- ¼ cup mushrooms
- ¼ cup tomatoes

DIRECTIONS

1. In a bowl combine all ingredients together
2. In a pan heat olive oil and pour the mixture
3. Cook for 1-2 minutes per side
4. When ready sprinkle salt, pepper and serve

Serves: *1*
Prep Time: *5*   Minutes

Cook Time: *5*   Minutes

Total Time: *10*   Minutes

INGREDIENTS

- 2 eggs
- pinch of salt
- black pepper
- ¼ cup cheese
- olive oil

DIRECTIONS

1. In a bowl combine all ingredients together
2. In a skillet heat oil
3. Pour mixture and cook for 1-2 minutes per side
4. When ready remove from heat and serve

Serves: *1*

Prep Time: **5** Minutes

Cook Time: **5** Minutes

Total Time: *10* Minutes

INGREDIENTS

- 3 oz. cheddar cheese
- 2 slices ham
- 2 eggs
- 1 tablespoon basil
- Pinch of salt
- olive oil

DIRECTIONS

1. In a bowl combine all ingredients together
2. In a skillet heat oil
3. Pour mixture and cook for 1-2 minutes per side
4. When ready remove from heat and serve

Serves: *1*
Prep Time: **5**   Minutes

Cook Time: **5**   Minutes

Total Time: **10**   Minutes

INGREDIENTS

- 2 eggs
- 1/4 cup spinach
- ¼ onion
- ¼ tomato
- olive oil
- pinch of salt

DIRECTIONS

1. In a bowl combine all ingredients together
2. In a skillet heat oil
3. Pour mixture and cook for 1-2 minutes per side
4. When ready remove from heat and serve

STEAK AND PEPPER

Serves: *4*
Prep Time: *10*   Minutes

Cook Time: *20*   Minutes

Total Time: *30*   Minutes

INGREDIENTS

- ¼ tsp salt
- ¼ tsp pepper
- 1 lb. beef
- 2 cloves garlic
- 1 pepper
- 1 onion
- 1 tsp sugar
- ¼ cup coffee
- ¼ cup vinegar
- 2 cups watercress
- olive oil

DIRECTIONS

1. In a bowl combine all seasoning together and rub steak with the mixture

2. In a skillet heat olive oil, add the steak and cook for 4-5 minutes per side

3. When ready transfer to a cutting board

4. In the skillet add onion, bell peppers, coffee, vinegar and cook for 4-5 minutes

5. When ready serve steak with watercress and sautéed peppers

Serves: *6*

Prep Time: *8*   Hours

Cook Time: *1*   Hours

Total Time: *9*   Hours

INGREDIENTS

- ¼ cup orange juice
- 2 lb. chicken breast
- 1 tablespoon olive oil
- 1 tablespoon ginger
- 1 tsp paprika
- ¼ tsp red pepper
- ¼ tsp salt
- 1 tsp orange peel
- 1 tablespoon honey
- 1 tsp orange juice

DIRECTIONS

1. In a plastic bag add the chicken and marinade
2. For the marinade combine in a bowl olive oil, paprika, orange juice, red pepper and salt

3. Let the chicken marinade overnight

4. In a bowl combine orange juice and honey

5. Grill the chicken for 50-60 minutes at 175 F and brush
   with honey mixture while grilling

6. When ready remove and serve

Serves: *6*

Prep Time: *10*   Minutes

Cook Time: *30*   Minutes

Total Time: *40*   Minutes

INGREDIENTS

- 6 oz. turkey sausage
- 1 tsp olive oil
- ¼ scallions
- ¼ cup swiss cheese
- 4 eggs
- 2 egg whites
- 1 tsp pepper
- 1 cup milk

DIRECTIONS

1. Preheat the oven to 300 F

2. In a skillet cook sausage and mushrooms until golden brown

3. Stir in cheese, pepper and scallions

4. Whisk egg whites, eggs, milk and divide egg mixture among each muffin cups

5. Add sausage mixture and bake for 25-30 minutes or until golden brown

6. When ready remove and serve

Serves: *8*

Prep Time: *5*   Minutes

Cook Time: *10*   Minutes

Total Time: *15*   Minutes

INGREDIENTS

- 1 tsp lemon zest
- 1 tsp rosemary
- 1 tsp olive oil
- 2 cloves garlic
- ¼ tsp salt
- ¼ tsp pepper
- 1 lb. salmon
- Cherry tomatoes

DIRECTIONS

1. In a bowl combine oil, lemon zest, salt, garlic and pepper
2. Add salmon, toss to coat and divide the salmon among 8-10 skewers

3. Grill the skewers for 5-6 minutes or the salmon is
    done

4. When ready remove and serve

Serves: *2*
Prep Time: *10*   Minutes

Cook Time: *50*   Minutes

Total Time: *60*   Minutes

INGREDIENTS

- 1 lb. tomatoes
- 1 onion
- 1 tablespoon orange zest
- 1 tsp olive oil
- 1 tablespoon thyme leaves
- 1 lb. cod fish
- 2-4 springs thyme

DIRECTIONS

1. In a bowl combine orange zest, tomatoes, thyme and onions
2. Place the fish in the marinade and sprinkle salt and pepper while marinating
3. Roast for 40-50 minutes at 425 F
4. When ready remove from the oven and serve

Serves: *4*
Prep Time: *10*   Minutes

Cook Time: *20*   Minutes

Total Time: *30*   Minutes

INGREDIENTS

- 1 lb. lean tenderloin pork
- 1 tsp oil
- ¼ cup apple cider
- 1 tsp vinegar
- 1 tsp chili powder
- ¼ tsp chipotle chile

DIRECTIONS

1. In a bowl combine salt, chili powder and sprinkle pork with the mixture
2. In a skillet heat oil and add the pork, cook until golden brown on each side
3. Add vinegar, cider and bring to a boil
4. Reduce heat and cook for another 2-3 minutes
5. When ready serve pork with the glaze

Serves: **6**

Prep Time: **10** Minutes

Cook Time: **20** Minutes

Total Time: **30** Minutes

INGREDIENTS

- 1 cup broth
- 2 tomatoes
- 1 cups rice
- ½ cup basil
- 1 cup cheese

DIRECTIONS

1. In a skillet cook sausage for 5-6 minutes
2. Stir in broth, tomatoes, rice and simmer on low heat for 8-10 minutes
3. Stir in cheese, rice, basil and divide the filling among the peppers
4. Top with more cheese and cook until is melted
5. Serve when ready

Serves: *4*

Prep Time: *10*   Minutes

Cook Time: *20*   Minutes

Total Time: *30*   Minutes

INGREDIENTS

- 2 tablespoons lemon juice
- 2 tablespoons wine
- 1 tsp olive oil
- 2 cloves garlic
- 1 lb. shrimp
- 1 bay leaf
- ½ tsp red pepper
- ½ tsp salt
- 1 tablespoon parsley

DIRECTIONS

1. In a bowl combine garlic, oil and lemon juice
2. Add shrimp and marinade for 20-30 minutes
3. In a skillet heat olive oil, add shrimp and cook for 1-2 minutes per side

4. Add red pepper, bay leaf, used marinade and simmer
    for 4-5 minutes

5. Sprinkle with parsley salt and cook until the shrimp
    is ready

Serves: *6*
Prep Time: *10*   Minutes

Cook Time: *15*   Minutes

Total Time: *25*   Minutes

INGREDIENTS

- 1 tsp oil
- 1 shallot
- 1 lb. beans
- ¼ cup water
- 1 slice bacon
- 1 tablespoon nuts
- ½ tsp salt

DIRECTIONS

1. In a skillet add shallot and cook for 1-2 minutes
2. Add green beans and cook for 4-5 minutes
3. Add water, reduce heat and cook for 6-8 minutes
4. Remove from heat, stir in bacon and salt
5. When ready remove from heat and serve

Serves: **6**

Prep Time: **10**   Minutes

Cook Time: **67**   Minutes

Total Time: **40**   Minutes

INGREDIENTS

- **1 tablespoon olive oil**
- **1 onion**
- **1 cup rice**
- **2 cloves garlic**
- **25 oz. chicken broth**
- **6 oz. asparagus**
- **1 cup peas**
- **¼ cup wine**
- **1 cup peppers**
- **1 cup parmesan cheese**
- **¼ cup chives**
- **1 tsp lemon zest**

DIRECTIONS

1. **In a Dutch oven add onions and cook until soft**

2. Stir in garlic, rice, wine and simmer until wine has evaporated

3. Add broth and cover the pan

4. Bake the rice at 400 F for 60 minutes

5. Steam asparagus, bell pepper and peas for 5-6 minutes

6. Add parsley, chives, vegetables, lemon zest and pepper into the risotto

7. Serve when ready

Serves: *6*

Prep Time: *10*   Minutes

Cook Time: *30*   Minutes

Total Time: *40*   Minutes

INGREDIENTS

- 1 lb. potatoes
- 1 cup olive oil
- 1 tsp rosemary
- ¼ tsp salt
- 2 tomatoes
- 2 cloves garlic
- ½ cup Parmesan cheese

DIRECTIONS

1. Preheat the oven to 425 F
2. In a bowl combine rosemary, salt, pepper and drizzle over potatoes
3. Bake for 20 minutes or until golden brown
4. Add garlic, olives, tomatoes and bake for another 10 minutes

5. When ready transfer to a dish and serve with parmesan cheese

Serves: *4*

Prep Time: *15*   Minutes

Cook Time: *35*   Minutes

Total Time: *50*   Minutes

INGREDIENTS

- 1 lb. chicken thigs
- 1 tablespoon olive oil
- 1 carrot
- 2 cans chicken broth
- 1 cup water
- 1 tablespoon vinegar
- 1 tablespoon soy sauce
- 2 tsp ginger
- 3 oz. rice noodles
- 4 oz. pea pods

DIRECTIONS

1. In a Dutch oven cook until golden brown
2. Add broth, water, carrots, vinegar, ginger, soy sauce, bring to a boil and simmer for 15-20 minutes

3. Add noodles, simmer for 5-10 minutes and then add
    pea pods

4. When ready remove from heat and serve

Serves: *1*
Prep Time: *5*   Minutes

Cook Time: *5*   Minutes

Total Time: *10*   Minutes

INGREDIENTS

- 1 head cauliflower
- ½ cup coconut milk
- Salt
- 1/3 cup chives

DIRECTIONS

1. Steam the cauliflower
2. When ready place the cauliflower in a blender and blend until smooth
3. Stir in salt, herbs, coconut milk, chives and blend again
4. Serve when ready

Serves: *2*

Prep Time: *10* Minutes

Cook Time: *35* Minutes

Total Time: *45* Minutes

INGREDIENTS

- 2 salmon fillets
- ¼ cup olive oil
- ¼ cup lemon juice
- salt

DIRECTIONS

1. Preheat the oven to 325 F
2. Marinade the salmon overnight
3. When ready sprinkle salmon with olive oil and salt
4. Bake for 30-35 minutes at 325 F or until the salmon is cooked
5. Add lemon juice and serve

Serves: *1*

Prep Time: *5*   Minutes

Cook Time: *5*   Minutes

Total Time: *10*   Minutes

INGREDIENTS

- ¼ cup zucchini
- ¼ cup red capsicum
- ½ cup yellow capsicum
- 1 cup sprouted moong
- ¼ cup apple
- 1 tablespoon olive oil
- 1 tsp lemon juice

DIRECTIONS

1. In a bowl combine all ingredients together
2. Add olive oil, toss well and serve

Serves: **1**

Prep Time: **5** Minutes

Cook Time: **5** Minutes

Total Time: **10** Minutes

INGREDIENTS

- ¼ cooked quinoa
- ¼ cup avocado
- ¼ cup zucchini
- ¼ cup capsicum cubes
- ¼ cup mushroom
- ½ cup cherry tomatoes
- 1 cup lettuce
- 1 tablespoon sprouts
- 1 tsp olive oil
- Salad dressing

DIRECTIONS

1. In a bowl combine all ingredients together
2. Add salad dressing, toss well and serve

Serves: *1*
Prep Time: *5*   Minutes

Cook Time: *5*   Minutes

Total Time: *10*   Minutes

INGREDIENTS

- ¼ mint leaves
- 2 cups apple cubes
- 1 tsp lemon juice
- 1 tsp ginger
- 1 tsp honey
- salt

DIRECTIONS

1. In a bowl combine all ingredients together
2. Add salad dressing, toss well and serve

Serves: **1**

Prep Time: **5** Minutes

Cook Time: **5** Minutes

Total Time: **10** Minutes

INGREDIENTS

- 1 cup avocados
- 1 cup tomatoes

SALAD DRESSING

- 1 tablespoon olive oil
- ¼ tsp mustard
- 1 tsp lemon juice
- salt

DIRECTIONS

1. In a bowl combine all ingredients together
2. Add salad dressing, toss well and serve

Serves: *1*
Prep Time: **5**   Minutes

Cook Time: **5**   Minutes

Total Time: **10**   Minutes

INGREDIENTS

- **2 cups bean sprouts**
- **¼ cup dill leaves**
- **¼ cup tomatoes**
- **1 tablespoon lemon juice**
- **¼ cup basil**
- **Salad dressing**

DIRECTIONS

1. **In a bowl combine all ingredients together**
2. **Add salad dressing, toss well and serve**

Serves: *1*

Prep Time: *5*   Minutes

Cook Time: *5*   Minutes

Total Time: *10*   Minutes

INGREDIENTS

- ¼ cup masoor
- ¼ cup cucumber
- ½ cup carrot
- ¼ cup tomatoes
- ¼ cup onion

SALAD DRESSING

- ¼ tablespoon olive oil
- 1 tsp lemon juice
- ¼ tsp green chillies
- ½ tsp black pepper

DIRECTIONS

1. In a bowl combine all ingredients together
2. Add salad dressing, toss well and serve

Serves: *1*
Prep Time: **5**   Minutes

Cook Time: **5**   Minutes

Total Time: *10*   Minutes

INGREDIENTS

- 1 cup muskmelon
- ½ cup pear cubes
- ½ cup apple cubes
- Salad dressing

DIRECTIONS

1. In a bowl combine all ingredients together
2. Add salad dressing, toss well and serve

Serves: *1*

Prep Time: *5*   Minutes

Cook Time: *5*   Minutes

Total Time: *10*   Minutes

INGREDIENTS

- 2 cups watermelon
- ¼ cup orange
- ¼ cup sweet lime
- ¼ cup pomegranate

SALAD DRESSING

- 1 tsp olive oil
- 1 tsp lemon juice
- 1 tablespoon parsley

DIRECTIONS

1. In a bowl combine all ingredients together
2. Add salad dressing, toss well and serve

Serves: *1*

Prep Time: *5*   Minutes

Cook Time: *5*   Minutes

Total Time: *10*   Minutes

INGREDIENTS

- 1 cup carrot
- 1 cup cucumber
- ¼ cup boiled rajma
- ¼ cup onions

SALAD DRESSING

- 1 tablespoon mint leaves
- 2 tsp honey
- 1 tablespoon lemon juice

DIRECTIONS

1. In a bowl combine all ingredients together
2. Add salad dressing, toss well and serve

Serves: **4**

Prep Time: **10**   Minutes

Cook Time: **30**   Minutes

Total Time: **40**   Minutes

INGREDIENTS

- 1 tablespoon mint leaves
- 1 cup chooked chawli
- ¼ cup cucumber
- ¼ cup onion
- ¼ cup tomatoes
- 1 tablespoon coriander
- ¼ tsp green chillies

SALAD DRESSING

- ¼ tsp salt
- ¼ tablespoon lemon juice
- ¼ tsp olive oil

DIRECTIONS

1. In a bowl combine all ingredients together
2. Add salad dressing, toss well and serve

BARLEY SOUP

Serves: *2*

Prep Time: *10*   Minutes

Cook Time: *20*   Minutes

Total Time: *30*   Minutes

INGREDIENTS

- 1 tablespoon barley
- 1 tsp oil
- 1 tsp garlic
- ¼ cup spring onions whites
- ¼ cup carrots
- 1 tablespoon red lentil
- ¼ cup tomatoes
- ¼ cup onion greens
- 1 tablespoon coriander

DIRECTIONS

1. In a pressure cooker add garlic, onion whites and sauté

2. Add masoor, barley, carrots, water, salt and cook for
    another 4-5 minutes

3. Allow to steam and transfer mixture to a pan

4. Add the rest of the ingredients and boil for 3-4
    minutes

5. When ready remove from heat and serve

Serves: *4*

Prep Time: *10*   Minutes

Cook Time: *3*   Hours

Total Time: *3*   Hours 10 Minutes

INGREDIENTS

- 2 cups sprouts
- ¼ cup mint leaves
- 1 cup tomatoes
- ¼ cup onions
- 1 tablespoon garlic
- salt
- 1 tablespoon lemon juice

DIRECTIONS

1. In a pressure cooker add sprouts, onion, garlic, tomatoes, water and cook for 2-3 hours
2. Cook until the vegetables are tender and water partially evaporated
3. Blend the soup and transfer the mixture to a pan

4. Add salt, mint leaves and cook for another 4-5
    minutes

5. When ready remove from heat and serve

Serves: *4*

Prep Time: *10*   Minutes

Cook Time: *3*   Hours

Total Time: *3*   Hours 10 Minutes

INGREDIENTS

- ½ cup masoor dal
- ¼ cup mint leaves
- ½ cup onions
- ½ cup carrot
- ½ cup tomatoes
- ¼ tsp red chilli flakes
- salt

DIRECTIONS

1. In a pan add mint leaves and roast for 2-3 minutes
2. In a pressure cooker add masoor, carrot, tomatoes, onions, water and cook for 2-3 hours
3. When ready allow to cool and blend the soup
4. Transfer to the pan with the mint leaves and cook for 4-5 minutes

Serves: *4*

Prep Time: *10*   Minutes

Cook Time: *40*   Minutes

Total Time: *50*   Minutes

INGREDIENTS

- 2 tablespoons oil
- 2 tsp garlic
- ¼ tsp black peppercorns
- ½ cup tomatoes
- 3 cups vegetable stock
- ½ cup zucchini
- ½ cup carrots
- 1 tsp celery
- 2 tablespoons parsley

DIRECTIONS

1. In a pan add onion, garlic and sauté for 2-3 minutes
2. Add black peppercorns, salt, tomatoes and sauté for 2-3 minutes
3. Add vegetable stock and bring to a boil

4. Add celery, carrots, zucchini and simmer for 30 minutes

5. When ready add parsley mix well and serve

Serves: *4*

Prep Time: *10*   Minutes

Cook Time: *25*   Minutes

Total Time: *35*   Minutes

INGREDIENTS

- 1 tablespoon olive oil
- 1 onion
- 1 lb. carrot
- 1 tablespoon garam masala
- Juice ½ orange
- 1 L vegetable stock
- 200ml coconut milk
- 1 lb. mixed beans

DIRECTIONS

1. In a saucepan cook carrots and onions until soft
2. Add ginger, garam masala and cook for 2-3 minutes
3. Add stock, orange juice and simmer for 12-15 minutes
4. Transfer soup to a blender and blend until smooth
5. Add beans and blend again

6. Transfer soup back to a saucepan and cook for another 3-4 minutes

7. When ready remove from heat and serve

Serves: *4*
Prep Time: *10*   Minutes

Cook Time: *25*   Minutes

Total Time: *35*   Minutes

INGREDIENTS

- 1 tablespoon olive oil
- 1 lb. leeks
- 1 lb. courgettes
- 2 tsp bouillon
- 1 lb. spinach
- ¼ lb. goat cheese
- 1 oz. basil

DIRECTIONS

1. In a pan fry leek, add courgettes and cook for 4-5 minutes
2. Add stock, spinach, bouillon and cook for 12-15 minutes
3. Blend the soup, add cheese and blend again
4. Serve when ready

Serves: *4*

Prep Time: *10*   Minutes

Cook Time: *30*   Minutes

Total Time: *40*   Minutes

INGREDIENTS

- 1 oz. butter
- 1 lb. asparagus spear
- 2 shallots
- 2 garlic coves
- 2 handfuls of spinach
- 1 L vegetable stock
- olive oil

DIRECTIONS

1. In a saucepan fry asparagus until soft
2. Add garlic, shallots and cook for 8-10 minutes
3. Stir in spinach, stock and bring to a boil
4. Cook until most of the liquid evaporated
5. Transfer soup to a blender and blend until smooth
6. When ready season soup and serve

Serves: *4*

Prep Time: *10*   Minutes

Cook Time: *25*   Minutes

Total Time: *35*   Minutes

INGREDIENTS

- 1 tsp olive oil
- 1 cucumber
- 1 lettuce
- ½ lb. peas
- 2 tsp bouillon
- Large bun of spring onions
- 1L water

DIRECTIONS

1. In a frying pan cook onion for 4-5 minutes, add lettuce, peas, cucumber and pour over boiling water
2. Stir in bouillon and simmer for 12-15 minutes
3. When vegetables are soft transfer soup to a blender and blend
4. Serve when ready

Serves: *4*
Prep Time: *10*   Minutes

Cook Time: *40*   Minutes

Total Time: *50*   Minutes

INGREDIENTS

- 2 tablespoons olive oil
- 1 lb. celery
- 1 garlic clove
- ½ lb. potatoes
- 500 ml vegetable stock
- 100 ml milk

DIRECTIONS

1. In a saucepan add potatoes, garlic, celery, water, salt and cook for 15-18 minutes
2. Add vegetable stock and bring to a boil, simmer for 15-20 minutes
3. When ready blend the soup, season and serve

Serves: *5*

Prep Time: *10*   Minutes

Cook Time: *20*   Minutes

Total Time: *30*   Minutes

INGREDIENTS

- ¼ cup barley
- ½ cup moong dal
- 1 cup bottle gourd
- 1 cup carrot
- ¼ tablespoon carrot
- 1 tsp cumin seeds
- 2 peppercorns
- 1 bay leaf
- 2 cloves
- ¼ tsp turmeric powder

DIRECTIONS

1. In a pressure cooker add cumin seeds, peppercorns, bay leaf, cloves and sauté for 1-2 minutes

2. Add carrot, barley, moong dal, turmeric, salt, water,
    and cook until the vegetables are soft

3. When ready remove and serve

Serves: **2**

Prep Time: **10**   Minutes

Cook Time: **35**   Minutes

Total Time: **45**   Minutes

INGREDIENTS

- 2 cups carrots
- 2 cups fenugreek
- ¼ tsp cumin seeds
- ¼ cup onions
- 2 green chillies
- 1 clove
- 1-piece ginger
- ¼ tsp turmeric powder
- 1 tsp coriander
- 1 tsp olive oil

DIRECTIONS

1. In a pan heat olive and add cumin seeds
2. Add green chillies, onions, ginger and sauté for 2-3 minutes

3. Add carrots, fenugreek, coriander, turmeric powder, salt, water and cook on low until liquid has evaporated

4. When vegetables are tender remove from heat and serve

Serves: 2
Prep Time: 5   Minutes

Cook Time: 25   Minutes

Total Time: 35   Minutes

INGREDIENTS

- ¼ cup toovar
- ¼ cup moong dal
- ¼ cup chana dal
- 1 cup fenugreek
- 1 cup coriander
- ½ cup green peas
- ½ cup coconut
- 2 green chillies
- ¼ cup onions
- ¼ cup carrot
- salt

DIRECTIONS

1. Soak the dals in water for 2-3 hours

2. Grind dals to paste, add the rest of the ingredients and mix well

3. Steam the paste for 12-15 minutes or until everything is tender

4. When ready remove from heat and serve

Serves: **2**

Prep Time: **5**   Minutes

Cook Time: **20**   Minutes

Total Time: **25**   Minutes

INGREDIENTS

- ½ cup cucumber
- ½ cup chana dal
- 1 tsp cumin seeds
- ½ tsp chili powder
- 1 tsp turmeric powder
- 1 tsp olive oil

DIRECTIONS

1. Soak the chana dal in water for 1-2 hours
2. In a pan add cumin seeds and sauté for 1-2 minutes
3. Add the rest of the ingredients in the pan and cook for 12-15 minutes
4. When ready remove from heat and serve

Serves: **4**

Prep Time: **10**   Minutes

Cook Time: **30**   Minutes

Total Time: **40**   Minutes

INGREDIENTS

- ¼ cup oats
- ½ cup cooked brown rice
- 1 tablespoon moong dal
- 1 tsp olive oil
- ¼ cup onions
- 1 tsp garlic
- ¼ tsp ginger
- ½ cup beans
- ¼ cup carrot
- ¼ cup green peas
- 1 tablespoon coriander

DIRECTIONS

1. **In a pressure cooker add onions, garlic, ginger and sauté for 2-3 minutes**

2. Add green peas, beans, carrot and sauté for another 2-3 minutes

3. Add the rest of the ingredients, water and cook for another 5-6 minutes

4. Cook until the water has evaporated

5. When ready remove from heat and serve

Serves: *1*

Prep Time: **5**   Minutes

Cook Time: **5**   Minutes

Total Time: ***10***   Minutes

INGREDIENTS

- 1 cup avocado
- 1 tsp lemon juice
- 1 tablespoon tomatoes
- ¼ tsp green chillies
- salt

DIRECTIONS

1. In a blender combine all ingredients together
2. Blend until smooth
3. When ready remove and serve

Serves: 2

Prep Time: 5   Minutes

Cook Time: 20   Minutes

Total Time: 25   Minutes

INGREDIENTS

- ½ cup buckwheat
- ½ cup sprouts
- ½ cup moong dal
- 1 tsp olive oil
- 1 black peppercorn
- ¼ tsp cumin seeds
- 2 cloves
- ¼ tsp turmeric powder

DIRECTIONS

1. In a pressure cooker add cloves, cumin seeds and peppercorn, sauté for 2-3 minutes
2. Add the rest of the ingredients and water
3. Simmer for 12-15 minutes or until vegetables are soft
4. When ready remove from heat and serve

Serves: *4*

Prep Time: *10*   Minutes

Cook Time: *40*   Minutes

Total Time: *50*   Minutes

INGREDIENTS

- 1 cup brown rice
- Salt
- 1 tsp olive oil

DIRECTIONS

1. Soak the brown rice in water for 30-40 minutes
2. When ready transfer to a pressure cooker
3. Cook for 6 whistles, when ready remove and serve

CARROT DRINK

Serves: *1*

Prep Time: *5*   Minutes

Cook Time: *5*   Minutes

Total Time: *10*   Minutes

INGREDIENTS

- 2 cups carrots
- 1 cup apple
- ½ tsp brown sugar

DIRECTIONS

1. In a blender place all ingredients and blend until smooth
2. Pour smoothie in a glass and serve

Serves: *1*

Prep Time: **5**   Minutes

Cook Time: **5**   Minutes

Total Time: **10**   Minutes

INGREDIENTS

- **2 cups watermelon**
- **¼ cup tomatoes**
- **¼ cup apples**
- **¼ cup pears**

DIRECTIONS

1. **In a blender place all ingredients and blend until smooth**
2. **Pour smoothie in a glass and serve**

Serves: *1*
Prep Time: **5**   Minutes

Cook Time: **5**   Minutes

Total Time: ***10***   Minutes

INGREDIENTS

- 2 cups muskmelon
- 2 cups pineapple
- 1 cup ice

DIRECTIONS

1. In a blender place all ingredients and blend until smooth
2. Pour smoothie in a glass and serve

Serves: *1*

Prep Time: *5*   Minutes

Cook Time: *5*   Minutes

Total Time: *10*   Minutes

INGREDIENTS

- 1 cup carrot
- 1 cup beetroot
- 1 tablespoon parsley
- 1 tablespoon celery
- 1 cup ice

DIRECTIONS

1. In a blender place all ingredients and blend until smooth
2. Pour smoothie in a glass and serve

Serves: *1*
Prep Time: 5   Minutes

Cook Time: 5   Minutes

Total Time: *10*   Minutes

INGREDIENTS

- 1 cup watermelon
- 1-piece ginger
- 1 cup ice
- 1 cup melon

DIRECTIONS

1. **In a blender place all ingredients and blend until smooth**
2. **Pour smoothie in a glass and serve**

Serves: *1*
Prep Time: *5*   Minutes

Cook Time: *5*   Minutes

Total Time: *10*   Minutes

INGREDIENTS

- ½ cup papaya cubes
- ½ cup coconut
- ½ cup coconut water
- 1 cup ice

DIRECTIONS

1. In a blender place all ingredients and blend until smooth
2. Pour smoothie in a glass and serve

Serves: *1*

Prep Time: *5*   Minutes

Cook Time: *5*   Minutes

Total Time: *10*   Minutes

INGREDIENTS

- 1 cup red capsicum
- 1 cup carrot
- 1 cup apple
- 1 cup ice

DIRECTIONS

1. **In a blender place all ingredients and blend until smooth**
2. **Pour smoothie in a glass and serve**

Serves: *1*
Prep Time: *5*   Minutes

Cook Time: *5*   Minutes

Total Time: *10*   Minutes

INGREDIENTS

- 1 tablespoon tyrosine
- ½ cup kale
- ½ cup watercress
- ¼ cup spinach
- ¼ cup antioxidants
- 1 cup ice

DIRECTIONS

1. In a blender place all ingredients and blend until smooth
2. Pour smoothie in a glass and serve

85

Serves: *1*

Prep Time: **5**   Minutes

Cook Time: **5**   Minutes

Total Time: ***10***   Minutes

INGREDIENTS

- **2 nuts**
- **2 stems cilantro**
- **1 pear**
- **1 orange**
- **2 tablespoons pumpkin seeds**
- **¼ cup yogurt**

DIRECTIONS

1. **In a blender place all ingredients and blend until smooth**
2. **Pour smoothie in a glass and serve**

Serves: *1*

Prep Time: *5* Minutes

Cook Time: *5* Minutes

Total Time: *10* Minutes

INGREDIENTS

- 1 banana
- 3 brazil nuts
- 350 ml unsweetened coconut milk
- 2 tablespoons cocoa powder
- 1 cup ice

DIRECTIONS

1. In a blender place all ingredients and blend until smooth
2. Pour smoothie in a glass and serve